ARTHRITIS DISEASE

DIET COOKBOOK

Delicious Anti-Inflammatory Recipes For Joint Pain Relief, Reduced Swelling, And Improved Mobility

DR ELIAN GRIFFIN

Copyright © [Elian Griffin] [2024]. All rights reserved.

DISCLAIMER

The nutritional recommendations and recipes in this book are meant solely for informative reasons. They are not meant to replace the counsel, diagnosis, or care of a qualified medical expert. If you have any doubts about a medical condition or dietary requirements, you should always see your physician or another trained healthcare expert.

All reasonable efforts have been taken by the author and publisher to ensure that the information contained in this book is correct as of the date of publication. Recommendations may alter, though, as medical knowledge is always changing. When using any of the recipes or instructions found here, the user assumes all liability and assumes no risk, whether personal or otherwise. People who have certain dietary requirements or medical issues should speak with a healthcare provider for personalized guidance. The given recipes are only ideas; you may need to adjust them to suit your own nutritional needs, tastes, and tolerances.

When you use this book, you agree to release the publisher, the author, and their representatives from any liability for any claims, damages, liabilities, costs, or expenditures resulting from your use of the book.

TABLE OF CONTENTS

ABOUT THE BOOK

The "Arthritis Disease Diet Cookbook" is an invaluable resource for anyone attempting to manage the difficulties associated with arthritis. It highlights the critical role that nutrition plays in effectively managing this condition. It is important to comprehend arthritis and how it affects dietary choices because the diet is a major factor in symptom relief and joint health maintenance.

By emphasizing foods high in nutrients and making well-informed dietary choices, people may be able to decrease inflammation, manage pain, and improve their quality of life.

This cookbook has been painstakingly designed to provide readers with a thorough understanding of arthritis and its dietary implications. It describes the various forms of arthritis and their symptoms, illuminating how specific dietary choices can reduce these symptoms. It highlights the significance of a well-balanced diet and offers useful insights into how dietary choices affect arthritis symptoms, motivating readers to take an active role in their health.

Comprehensive chapters on vital nutrients essential for managing arthritis are a key feature of this cookbook; it highlights nutrients like antioxidants and omega-3 fatty acids, outlining their health benefits and suggesting sources to include in daily meals. Useful advice on meal planning, goal-setting, and preparing balanced meals accommodates a range of needs and tastes, guaranteeing accessibility and simplicity in adopting healthier eating practices.

Breakfast, lunch, dinner, snack, and dessert recipes are all geared toward providing joint health benefits while also being delicious and full of nutrition. From healthy smoothies to hearty one-pot meals and baking tips for people with arthritis, every recipe is thoughtfully created to support wellness without compromising flavor. Seasonal variations and inexpensive shopping tips round out the cookbook's practicality and help make healthy eating a reality in daily life.

Apart from recipes, the cookbook explores lifestyle strategies that are crucial for arthritis management in its entirety. It talks about how exercise contributes to joint health, how to effectively manage stress, and how sleep affects symptom management. It also offers helpful tips on how to incorporate mindfulness into everyday routines and navigate common dietary concerns like handling flare-ups, eating out, and managing weight. All of these topics enhance the reader's experience and provide them with holistic strategies for long-term health improvement.

With thorough FAQs that offer guidance on managing dietary restrictions, deciphering food labels, and modifying diets during flare-ups, this cookbook ensures that readers feel informed and supported throughout their journey. It is an invaluable resource for anyone looking to proactively manage arthritis through dietary and lifestyle modifications that promote long-term health and well-being.

CHAPTER ONE

ARTHRITIS DISEASE DIET INTRODUCTION

KNOWING ARTHRITIS AND HOW IT AFFECTS DIET

Millions of people worldwide suffer from osteoarthritis and rheumatoid arthritis, two conditions that cause joint pain, stiffness, and inflammation. Arthritis requires more than medication to treat; a comprehensive approach that includes dietary and lifestyle modifications is required. It is important to understand how arthritis affects diet to effectively manage symptoms.

Foods high in processed foods, refined sugars, and saturated fats can aggravate inflammation and make symptoms worse. On the other hand, a diet high in anti-inflammatory foods, such as fruits, vegetables, whole grains, and omega-3 fatty acids, can help reduce inflammation and ease pain. Knowledge of these dietary effects enables people to make decisions that promote joint health.

In addition to avoiding trigger foods, an arthritis-friendly diet should also make sure that the body gets enough of the nutrients that support joint function, such as antioxidants, vitamins C and D, and minerals like calcium and magnesium.

THE ROLE OF NUTRITION IN THE MANAGEMENT OF ARTHRITIS

A balanced diet specifically designed for people with arthritis can help reduce pain, stiffness, and swelling while improving joint function. Appropriate nutrition supports the immune system and helps maintain a healthy weight, which is crucial for reducing strain on joints affected by arthritis. Nutrition plays a pivotal role in managing arthritis by influencing inflammation levels, joint health, and overall well-being.

Anti-inflammatory foods: Including berries, nuts, fatty fish, and leafy greens in daily meals can help reduce the symptoms associated with arthritis. These foods are packed with nutrients and compounds that fight inflammation and support joint health. Staying hydrated: drinking lots of water helps lubricate joints and supports overall cellular function.

By putting nutrition first, people with arthritis can actively manage their symptoms and achieve better overall health outcomes. A nutritionally dense diet provides the building blocks for joint repair and maintenance, supporting long-term mobility and quality of life.

HOW YOU CAN USE THIS COOKBOOK TO HELP

This arthritis disease diet cookbook offers a range of recipes tailored to provide anti-inflammatory benefits while ensuring nutritional balance. All of the recipes are made with ingredients that are known to reduce inflammation and promote overall well-being. The cookbook is intended to make it easier to plan and prepare meals that support joint health and manage arthritis symptoms effectively.

This cookbook functions as a useful reference, providing simple-to-follow recipes that use common ingredients that are easily found in most grocery stores. Whether you're searching for hearty main courses, satisfying breakfast options, or healthy snacks, this cookbook offers a variety of meal ideas that suit a range of palates and dietary requirements. Nutritional data is included with each recipe to help you make educated diet choices.

This cookbook gives people the ability to take control of their diet in a way that enhances their quality of life and complements their medical treatment. It offers a wide variety of tasty and nutritious meals that support joint health and manage symptoms of arthritis.

SOME ADVICE FOR BEGINNING

A few helpful pointers will make starting an arthritis-friendly diet easier. To start, familiarize yourself with foods that support joint health and lower inflammation, like berries, leafy greens, and oily fish like salmon. Make sure your meals are planned ahead of time to include a variety of these beneficial foods while avoiding processed and sugary foods that exacerbate inflammation.

Try different flavors and meal combinations from the cookbook; gradually work these recipes into your weekly meal plans to get the most out of an arthritis-friendly diet. And don't forget to stay hydrated all day long by sipping herbal teas and water to help with joint lubrication and general hydration.

Consult a physician or dietitian to customize your diet plan according to your particular type of arthritis and your health objectives. They can offer customized guidance and recommendations to maximize your nutritional intake and promote your general health.

AN OVERVIEW OF FREQUENTLY USED INGREDIENTS

Many popular items with anti-inflammatory and nutritional benefits are used in this cookbook. Some of the main ingredients are:

• **Turmeric:** Frequently used to enhance food flavors and lessen joint discomfort, turmeric is well-known for its potent anti-inflammatory ingredient, curcumin.

• **Leafy Greens:** Packed with vitamins, minerals, and antioxidants, leafy greens like Swiss chard, spinach, and kale offer vital nutrients and support for joint health in general.

• **Berries:** Rich in vitamins and antioxidants, berries including raspberries, strawberries, and blueberries help fight inflammation and oxidative stress.

• **Oily Fish:** Omega-3 fatty acids, which are abundant in salmon, mackerel, and sardines, have anti-inflammatory qualities that may help lessen the symptoms of arthritis.

• **Nuts and Seeds:** Nutrients and good fats from almonds, walnuts, chia seeds, and flaxseeds enhance joint function and general health.

Try experimenting with different recipes to find combinations that suit your taste preferences and dietary needs.

CHAPTER TWO

WHAT IS AN INFLAMMATORY DISEASE?

Over 100 different types of joint diseases that cause pain, inflammation, stiffness, and swelling are collectively referred to as arthritis. Two of the most common types of arthritis are osteoarthritis (OA), which is caused by wear and tear on joints over time, resulting in cartilage breakdown and bone damage, and rheumatoid arthritis (RA), which is an autoimmune disorder where the immune system mistakenly attacks joint tissues, causing inflammation and potentially severe joint damage.

Joint pain, stiffness, and decreased range of motion are common symptoms of arthritis, which can have a major impact on daily life, mobility, and overall quality of life. Determining the type of arthritis one has is essential to creating a successful management plan, as lifestyle modifications and treatments can vary greatly depending on the particular condition.

DIFFERENT TYPES OF ARTHRITIS AND SYMPTOMS

Rheumatoid arthritis (RA), an autoimmune disease, causes inflammation that can damage joints and organs, frequently leading to swelling, joint deformity, and systemic symptoms like fatigue and fever.

Osteoarthritis (OA), the most common type of arthritis, usually affects older adults and results from the gradual breakdown of cartilage between joints, leading to pain and stiffness.

Other forms include psoriatic arthritis, which affects people with psoriasis and causes joint pain and inflammation; gout, which is characterized by sudden, severe attacks of pain, redness, and tenderness in joints due to uric acid crystal deposits; and juvenile arthritis, which affects children under the age of sixteen and comes in a variety of forms, each with its special challenges and symptoms.

Treatment regimens for arthritis frequently include medication, physical therapy, and lifestyle modifications intended to reduce pain, maintain joint function, and improve quality of life. Managing arthritis involves an accurate diagnosis as well as knowledge of the particular kind and its symptoms.

DIET'S FUNCTION IN MANAGING ARTHRITIS

A balanced diet rich in antioxidants, omega-3 fatty acids, and nutrients like vitamin D and calcium can support joint health and lessen the severity of symptoms. While no one diet can cure arthritis, making educated food choices can help reduce inflammation, manage weight, and improve overall well-being.

Some foods, like processed foods high in unhealthy fats and refined sugars, may make inflammation worse and should be avoided; anti-inflammatory foods, like nuts, fruits, and vegetables, can help reduce symptoms and promote general health; some people find relief by avoiding potential trigger foods, like nightshade vegetables or gluten, but the effects can differ greatly from person to person.

Speaking with a medical professional or registered dietitian can offer individualized advice on dietary changes based on personal requirements and preferences. People with arthritis may be able to lessen pain, improve joint function, and improve their overall quality of life by incorporating healthy eating habits into their daily lives.

THE VALUE OF A WELL-BALANCED DIET

A balanced diet provides essential nutrients that support joint health, such as vitamins, minerals, and antioxidants that help reduce inflammation and protect against joint damage. It also supports a healthy weight, which can lessen stress on joints and improve mobility. Maintaining a balanced diet is crucial for overall health and well-being, especially for people managing arthritis.

Lean proteins, whole grains, fruits, vegetables, and healthy fats are the main components of a balanced diet;

processed foods, sugar-filled drinks, and unhealthy fats should be avoided in excess as these can exacerbate arthritis symptoms and cause inflammation.

Hydration is also important, as adequate water intake helps maintain joint lubrication and overall cellular function. Nutrient-dense foods like leafy greens, berries, fatty fish, nuts, and seeds can provide antioxidants and omega-3 fatty acids that support joint health and reduce inflammation.

Through the adoption of a well-balanced diet customized to meet specific health needs and goals related to managing arthritis, people can maximize their nutritional intake, perhaps reduce symptoms, and improve their overall quality of life.

HOW DIETARY DECISIONS IMPACT ARTHRITIS SYMPTOMS

Food choices play a major role in arthritis symptoms and overall joint health. Depending on their nutritional makeup and how they interact with the body's inflammatory response, certain foods can either exacerbate inflammation or help alleviate symptoms. For example, foods high in unhealthy fats and refined sugars can promote inflammation, which in some people causes increased stiffness and pain in the joints.

On the other hand, if you include anti-inflammatory foods in your diet, like fatty fish (high in omega-3 fatty acids), nuts, seeds, and vibrant fruits and vegetables, you can help support joint health and lessen inflammation. These foods are packed with vital nutrients and antioxidants that help counteract oxidative stress and inflammation in the body.

Each person reacts differently to different foods, and some may find relief by avoiding possible trigger foods such as nightshade vegetables or gluten. Maintaining a food journal or consulting with a medical professional or qualified dietitian can assist in identifying individual dietary preferences and triggers.

CHAPTER THREE

CRUCIAL ELEMENTS FOR THE MANAGEMENT OF ARTHRITIS

AN OVERVIEW OF VITAL NUTRIENTS FOR THE MANAGEMENT OF ARTHRITIS

Important nutrients are important for controlling inflammation and maintaining joint health when managing arthritis through diet. Omega-3 fatty acids, which are abundant in fish (salmon, for example) and seeds (flaxseeds, for example) are well known for their anti-inflammatory qualities; these fats help relieve joint pain and stiffness by lowering the body's production of inflammatory chemicals. Antioxidants, which are present in colorful fruits and vegetables (berries, spinach, bell peppers, etc.), fight oxidative stress, which is one of the factors that causes joint damage in arthritis. Vitamins C and E, as well as minerals like selenium and zinc, also function as antioxidants, shielding joints from inflammation and damage.

A diverse range of nutrient-dense foods can greatly aid in the management of arthritis. Omega-3 fatty acids can be found in seafood such as salmon, mackerel, and sardines, while vegetarians can obtain their fill from plant-based sources like walnuts and chia seeds. Vibrantly colored fruits and vegetables like berries, cherries, spinach, and kale are full of antioxidants and vitamins that are important for joint health. Whole grains like brown rice and quinoa offer fiber and nutrients that support overall inflammation reduction. Lean proteins like chicken, tofu, and legumes provide the amino acids required for tissue repair and maintenance, which are vital for arthritis patients trying to preserve joint health.

RDAS (RECOMMENDED DAILY ALLOWANCES) FOR THE MANAGEMENT OF ARTHRITIS

To create a diet that is arthritis-friendly, one must be aware of the Recommended Daily Allowances (RDAs) for key nutrients. For example, the American Heart Association suggests getting your Omega-3 fatty acids from at least two servings of fatty fish per week or by taking fish oil supplements. Antioxidant-rich foods should be a part of every meal to meet your daily requirements for vitamins C and E, zinc, and selenium. A balanced intake of fruits, vegetables, whole grains, and lean proteins guarantees that arthritis patients get the nutrients they need to support joint function and reduce inflammation. A registered dietitian or healthcare provider can help customize RDAs based on an individual's age, health, and degree of arthritis symptoms.

NUTRITIONAL SUPPLEMENTS FOR THE TREATMENT OF ARTHRITIS

Supplements rich in Omega-3 fatty acids, such as fish oil, are highly recommended for their anti-inflammatory properties. Supplements containing chondroitin sulfate and glucosamine support joint structure and function, which may lessen pain and stiffness. Vitamin D supplements are essential for bone health and may help arthritis patients, especially those who have little sun exposure. It is important to speak with a healthcare provider before beginning any supplement regimen to make sure it is in line with your particular health needs and medication regimen.

INCLUDING SUPERFOODS IN YOUR DIET TO HELP WITH ARTHRITIS

Superfoods, renowned for their high nutrient content, can improve an arthritis-friendly diet. For example, the powerful anti-inflammatory properties of turmeric (curcumin) can help reduce arthritis symptoms when added to food or taken as a supplement. Berries, loaded with vitamins and antioxidants, can be consumed fresh, frozen, or blended into smoothies to support joint health. Leafy greens, like spinach and kale, offer essential vitamins and minerals, and nuts and seeds, like flaxseed and almonds, can promote heart health and reduce inflammation.

CHAPTER FOUR

MEAL PLANNING FOR ARTHRITIS DIET

CREATING DIETARY OBJECTIVES

The first step in effectively managing your arthritis symptoms through nutrition is to set specific goals, such as managing weight, reducing inflammation, or improving joint health. These goals should be reasonable, individualized, and based on your current health status and lifestyle, among other things. Consulting a healthcare provider or a nutritionist can help you define these goals more precisely.

Next, set quantifiable goals, like increasing your intake of anti-inflammatory foods like nuts, leafy greens, and fatty fish in your daily meals. Creating a schedule to reach these goals can give you direction and drive. For example, set a goal to attain a well-balanced, nutrient-dense diet within a given time frame. Monitoring your progress regularly and making necessary adjustments will guarantee that your dietary goals stay applicable and beneficial in the long run for managing your arthritis symptoms.

STRATEGIES FOR MEAL PLANNING

Maintaining a healthy and arthritis-friendly diet requires careful meal planning. To start, make a weekly meal plan that includes a range of foods high in vitamins, omega-3 fatty acids, and antioxidants. This will help to manage inflammation and support joint health. Make sure your meals are simple to make and make use of seasonal produce for maximum freshness and nutritional value.

To save time on busy days, think about batch cooking or preparing meals ahead of time. This will guarantee that you always have wholesome options on hand, which will lessen the likelihood that you will choose less healthful options. When planning meals, concentrate on including a variety of lean proteins, whole grains, fruits, and vegetables in each meal. This will guarantee that you receive a wide range of nutrients required for overall health and managing arthritis.

Finally, utilize technologies such as meal planner apps or web-based meal planners to expedite the planning process. These tools can create shopping lists, recommend recipes based on dietary requirements, and even compute the nutritional value per serving. By implementing these meal planning techniques, you can make eating a nutritious diet for arthritis easier while still enjoying tasty and filling meals.

MAKING WELL-COMPOSED MEALS

Meal planning is essential to maintaining joint health and effectively controlling the symptoms of arthritis. Begin by dividing your plate into quarters to guarantee a well-rounded meal: half of your plate should be devoted to fruits and vegetables, one quarter to lean proteins like fish or poultry, and the remaining quarter to whole grains or starchy vegetables. This method offers a variety of nutrients while keeping portion sizes under control.

A range of colors should be included in your meals because different colored fruits and vegetables have different health benefits. For example, dark leafy greens like spinach and kale are high in vitamins K and C, which support the immune system and bone health. Brightly colored berries have antioxidants that fight inflammation and promote joint health. Eating these foods regularly can help manage the symptoms of arthritis and enhance overall health.

Try enhancing the flavor of your meals with herbs, spices, and healthy fats like olive oil instead of depending too much on salt or saturated fats; these ingredients not only taste better, but they also have additional health benefits. By concentrating on making nutritious, delicious, and well-balanced meals, you can support your arthritis management goals while eating a varied and fulfilling diet.

CHANGING YOUR DIET IN RESPONSE TO SYMPTOMS OF ARTHRITIS

By tailoring your diet to individual challenges, you can modify your diet in response to your arthritis symptoms. To start, maintain a food journal to record any associations between your diet and flare-ups of symptoms. This information can be used to identify trigger foods, such as processed sugars, saturated fats, or nightshade vegetables, which may aggravate inflammation or joint pain.

Incorporating supplements like omega-3 fatty acids or turmeric can also provide additional support for managing inflammation and joint stiffness. Speaking with a registered dietitian or healthcare provider can offer personalized guidance on adjusting your diet to better manage arthritis symptoms. You may also want to think about eliminating or reducing these trigger foods while increasing your intake of anti-inflammatory foods like fatty fish, nuts, and seeds.

Try varying the diet a little at a time to see how it affects the severity of your symptoms and your overall quality of life. Small adjustments made over time can have a big impact on joint health and quality of life. By tailoring your diet plan to your specific needs and symptoms, you can effectively and sustainably manage your arthritis.

LOW-COST ADVICE FOR GROCERY AND DINNER PLANNING

Maintaining an arthritis-friendly diet without going over budget requires navigating a frugal approach to meal preparation and shopping. To start, plan your meals and make a shopping list based on your meal plan.

This will help you avoid impulsive purchases and make sure you only buy what you need, which will reduce food waste and save money.

To get the most out of your grocery budget, take advantage of seasonal produce and sales. Frozen fruits and vegetables are also less expensive than fresh produce while maintaining their nutritional value. When buying proteins, look for low-cost options like canned tuna or beans, which are high in protein and can be used in a variety of recipes.

Cook large portions of dishes like soups, stews, or casseroles that can be portioned and frozen for later use. This approach not only saves money but also ensures you always have nutritious meals on hand, reducing the temptation to opt for less healthy convenience foods. Batch cooking or preparing meals in bulk can further reduce costs and save time during busy weeks.

Finally, look for coupons or loyalty programs offered by grocery stores to further stretch your budget. By following these frugal shopping and meal preparation tips, you can maintain a healthy, arthritis-friendly diet without going over your means. Compare prices and consider shopping at discount stores or buying in bulk for staple items like grains, legumes, and cooking oils.

HEALTHY BREAKFAST SELECTIONS

A healthy breakfast can help you start the day off right. Whole grains, such as quinoa or oats, provide you with sustained energy and fiber. You can also top your oatmeal with fresh berries, which are high in antioxidants and known to reduce inflammation.

If you'd rather have something savory, try whole-grain toast with avocado and a poached egg, which provides healthy fats and protein that are essential for joint function.

If you're looking for a more nutrient-dense and refreshing way to start the day, smoothie bowls filled with spinach, berries, and a protein source like Greek yogurt or tofu are a great option. These options not only nourish your body but also help manage arthritis symptoms by reducing inflammation and supporting overall joint health. Greek yogurt with nuts and seeds is a great option for a lighter yet satisfying breakfast, as it offers calcium, protein, and omega-3 fatty acids that support bone health.

ENERGIZING JUICES AND SMOOTHIES

Refreshing smoothies and juices designed to support joint health can help you get through your mornings. For a tropical twist, blend pineapple, mango, and coconut water for hydration and anti-inflammatory properties.

Start with a green smoothie made of spinach, kale, and a splash of citrus juice for a burst of vitamins and antioxidants. Add a banana for creaminess and potassium, which helps maintain electrolyte balance, which is crucial for muscle and joint function.

If you're more of a juicer, try this colorful concoction of beets and berries that have been infused with ginger, which is known to have anti-inflammatory properties. Beetroot juice has nitrates that may enhance blood flow and lessen joint inflammation. On the other hand, a combination of carrot and orange juice that is high in beta-carotene and vitamin C supports the production of collagen, which is necessary for joint health. These invigorating beverages taste great and also help fight fatigue and promote general well-being, making them ideal additions to an arthritis-friendly diet.

IDEAS FOR A HEALTHY BRUNCH

Savor a savory vegetable frittata loaded with vibrant vegetables like bell peppers, spinach, and tomatoes, providing essential vitamins and minerals. For a fun brunch with friends and family, try these nutritious and delectable ideas: start with whole grain pancakes or waffles topped with fresh fruits like bananas and strawberries. Use whole grain flour for added fiber and nutrients, while fruits provide vitamins and antioxidants that promote joint health.

Try these whole grain wraps with lean protein (grilled chicken or tofu) and leafy greens and hummus for extra flavor and nutrition, or make a quinoa salad with cucumber, chickpeas, and lemon vinaigrette dressing for plant-based protein and fiber that promotes digestive health and lowers inflammation. These brunch ideas are not only delicious but also support joint function and inflammation reduction by combining nutrient-dense ingredients.

EASY AND QUICK RECIPES TO MAKE ON A BUSY MORNING

Make healthy muffins with whole grain flour, oats, and grated zucchini or carrots for extra nutrients and moisture. For hectic mornings, opt for quick and simple recipes that emphasize convenience without compromising on nutrition.

Overnight oats are a pantry staple that requires very little preparation time and comes in a myriad of flavor combinations. Toss oats with almond milk, chia seeds, and your preferred fruits or nuts, and let them soak overnight for a ready-to-eat breakfast full of fiber and antioxidants.

Another quick and simple recipe that will help you start your day right with balanced nutrition that supports joint health and overall well-being is smoothie packs. Simply prepare individual freezer bags filled with spinach, berries, and a protein source like Greek yogurt or protein powder. In the morning, simply blend with almond milk or coconut water for a nutritious and filling smoothie in minutes. For a savory twist, make-ahead breakfast burritos filled with scrambled eggs, black beans, and salsa wrapped in whole grain tortillas.

SOME ADVICE ON CREATING AN ARTHRITIS-FRIENDLY BREAKFAST

Simple suggestions to improve joint health and decrease inflammation can help make your morning more arthritis-friendly. Opt for whole grains such as quinoa, oats, or whole wheat bread to sustain energy and fiber without triggering blood sugar spikes. Include foods high in omega-3, like flaxseeds, walnuts, or chia seeds, in your meals to help support joint function and reduce inflammation.

Eat plenty of colorful fruits and vegetables high in antioxidants and vitamins C and E, which help combat oxidative stress and inflammation in the body; minimize processed foods and sugary snacks, as they can exacerbate inflammation and joint pain; and stay hydrated throughout the day by drinking plenty of water or herbal teas to support joint lubrication and overall hydration levels. These tips ensure a delicious breakfast that also supports your arthritis management goals. Lean protein sources, such as eggs, Greek yogurt, or tofu, are an excellent way to support muscle strength and repair, which is crucial for maintaining joint health.

WELL-PROPORTIONED LUNCHES FOR LONG-TERM ENERGY

Incorporating a range of nutrient-dense foods, such as lean proteins, whole grains, and plenty of colorful vegetables, is the first step toward creating balanced lunches that sustain energy throughout the day and help manage arthritis. For example, a balanced lunch might consist of grilled chicken breast with quinoa and a side of roasted vegetables, which provide protein for muscle repair, complex carbohydrates for long-lasting energy, and antioxidants to fight inflammation.

If you want to make preparation easier, think about prepping ingredients like grains and proteins in bulk at the start of the week. This way, you can make easy lunches every day without having to worry about having to start from scratch. You can also add healthy fats, like avocado or olive oil-based dressings, for flavor and benefits for joint health.

Portion control is also critical; use smaller dishes or containers to prevent overindulging, which can lead to weight gain and increased stress on joints. Try different recipes and modify them according to individual dietary requirements and taste preferences. By emphasizing well-balanced nutrition and effective meal preparation, you can maximize your energy levels and support the management of your arthritis all day long.

DELICIOUS DINNER IDEAS

Cooking tasty dinners that satisfy the needs of an arthritic can be a delightful and healthful experience for the joints. To begin, experiment with anti-inflammatory herbs and spices such as turmeric, ginger, and garlic; these add flavor and also help to relieve pain naturally and support general well-being.

For a filling supper, try baked salmon with a glaze made of turmeric and lemon juice, which is served with quinoa salad topped with fresh herbs and veggies. The omega-3 fatty acids in the salmon provide lubrication for joints, while the high-fiber quinoa helps to maintain healthy digestion and blood sugar levels.

Try baking, steaming, or sautéing to retain nutrients and flavors without adding too much fat or oil. Use seasonal fruits and vegetables to add diversity and optimize nutritional value. By emphasizing whole, fresh foods and including ingredients that are good for arthritis, you can have tasty dinners that promote joint health and general well-being.

ONE-POT DINNERS FOR EASE

For arthritis sufferers who want to cut down on cleanup time and simplify dinner preparation, one-pot recipes are a great option. They cook all the ingredients in one pot, which eliminates the need for numerous pots and dishes.

Hearty soups, stews, and casseroles that mix grains or legumes, protein, and vegetables are popular one-pot meal ideas. For instance, a vegetable and lentil soup prepared with aromatic herbs and spices offers a nourishing and nutrient-dense meal that supports joint health.

For added convenience, use pre-cut veggies and pre-cooked grains or beans. Use pressure cookers or slow cookers to save time and work while producing tender, flavorful results. One-pot meals allow you to cook more efficiently, reduce joint strain, and enjoy tasty, arthritis-friendly meals with ease.

ADVICE ON USING ARTHRITIS-FRIENDLY COOKING METHODS

Using ergonomic kitchen tools and appliances, like jar openers, easy-grip knives, and food processors, can help reduce joint strain and make meal preparation more enjoyable and manageable. To begin, arrange your ingredients and kitchen tools in a way that minimizes reaching and bending.

Reduce the amount of time you spend cutting and chopping by modifying recipes to call for chopped or pre-sliced items. Try stir-frying instead of standing and stirring as much; it takes less time and effort.

Make small adjustments and incorporate arthritis-friendly techniques into your cooking routine to enjoy meal preparation while minimizing discomfort and promoting joint health.

For example, use multi-function cookers or countertop electric grills that simplify cooking processes and minimize manual effort.

SEASONAL DIFFERENCES IN MEAL SCHEDULING

Meal planning that takes seasonal variations into account guarantees a year-round supply of fresh, nutrient-dense ingredients and a variety of flavors. Start by learning about seasonal produce and incorporating it into your meals; in the summer, for instance, go for light salads and grilled vegetables that are hydrating and refreshing.

Winter greens and seasonal root vegetables make for hearty soups and stews that are not only comforting but also a good source of vitamins and minerals that support joint health and immune system function.

Try using different seasonal herbs and spices to add taste without using too much salt or sugar. When you accept seasonal changes, you can eat a variety of nutrient-dense, health-promoting meals.

HEALTHY SNACK SUGGESTIONS

If you take the proper approach, finding satisfying and healthful snack ideas for managing arthritis can be simple. Choose snacks that are high in anti-inflammatory components like fiber, antioxidants, and omega-3 fatty acids. Some examples of such snacks are a handful of walnuts or almonds combined with fresh berries to provide a dose of healthy fats and antioxidants; Greek yogurt with a sprinkling of chia seeds provides calcium and protein, which are essential for bone health and muscle function; and sliced vegetables like carrots, cucumbers, and bell peppers with hummus provide vitamins, minerals, and fiber while keeping calories in check.

A more substantial snack would be whole grain crackers with slices of avocado and flaxseeds or turmeric. The avocado provides good monounsaturated fats, and the turmeric has anti-inflammatory qualities. Apple slices spread with almond butter and a little cinnamon is a sweet but healthy snack that provides fiber, good fats, and natural sweetness without added sugars. Including these snacks in your daily diet not only help manage arthritis but also fosters overall wellness because of their delicious flavors and well-balanced nutrition.

SIMPLE AND QUICK APPETIZERS

It can be fun and stress-free to whip up quick and simple appetizers that satisfy arthritis-friendly diets. Choose recipes that call for little to no chopping or preparation time. For example, you can make a Mediterranean-inspired appetizer platter with olives, cherry tomatoes, and feta cheese that is drenched in olive oil and topped with dried herbs.

This combination tastes great and provides healthy fats from the olive oil, which is known to have anti-inflammatory properties. Another quick option is smoked salmon which is rolled with cucumber slices and a dab of cream cheese. This dish delivers protein and omega-3 fatty acids in a cool bite-sized format.

One savory option is mini quinoa-stuffed peppers, filled with cooked quinoa mixed with diced vegetables and a touch of cheese, then baked until golden. These appetizers are not only delicious but also nutritious, making them ideal for gatherings or as a light meal option. By focusing on simple ingredients and easy preparation methods, you can create appetizers that are both arthritis-friendly and enjoyable for everyone. Sweet potato rounds are rich in vitamins and fiber, supporting joint health, and Greek yogurt adds protein and probiotics.

CARRY-ALONG SNACKS FOR ANY SITUATION

Making batches of homemade trail mix with nuts, seeds, and dried fruits such as cranberries or apricots is a great way to find portable snacks that are both convenient and appropriate for managing arthritis. These snacks offer a combination of healthy fats, protein, and antioxidants, making them perfect for maintaining energy levels throughout the day. Whole grain energy bars or balls made with oats, nut butter, and honey are another portable option that provides a balance of carbohydrates and protein for long-lasting satiety.

Prepare veggie sticks like celery, cucumber, and baby carrots along with a small container of hummus or guacamole for dipping. These snacks are convenient for travel and can be enjoyed on their own or as part of a balanced meal. By planning and choosing nutritious options, you can maintain a healthy diet while on the go, promoting joint health and overall well-being. For a cool snack, pack pre-cut fruit like watermelon or pineapple in a container or zip-top bag. These fruits are hydrating and rich in vitamins and minerals, supporting overall health and joint function.

WHOLESOME SPREADS AND DIPS

An arthritis-friendly diet can be complemented with nutrient-dense, anti-inflammatory dips and spreads. To begin, try a classic guacamole, which is made from mashed ripe avocados with diced tomatoes, lime juice, and cilantro. Avocados are high in potassium and monounsaturated fats, which are good for the heart and muscles. Serve this guacamole with whole grain tortilla chips or vegetable crudités for a filling snack or appetizer. Alternatively, make homemade hummus with chickpeas, tahini, lemon juice, and garlic, which provides protein, fiber, and important minerals like iron and magnesium.

Try making a creamy almond butter dip for a dairy-free spread by combining almond butter with a little coconut milk, honey, or maple syrup. This dip goes well with fruit slices, whole grain crackers, or as a spread on toast. It offers natural sweetness and healthy fats without the need for added sugars.

You can also experiment with different herbs and spices like turmeric, ginger, or paprika to add flavor and anti-inflammatory properties to your spreads and dips. You can enjoy tasty flavors and promote joint health and overall wellness by incorporating these homemade creations into your meals and snacks.

An arthritis-friendly diet must control cravings without sacrificing health. When you have a craving for something salty or sweet, try these healthy substitutes: air-popped popcorn seasoned with a dash of nutritional yeast or herbs like rosemary and thyme; popcorn is a whole grain that's high in fiber and makes a filling snack that can help reduce hunger and cravings; if you have a sweet tooth, indulge in dark chocolate squares with a high cocoa content; these provide antioxidants and, when consumed in moderation, may have anti-inflammatory properties.

When you're in the mood for something creamy, try a smoothie made with Greek yogurt, frozen berries, spinach, and a dollop of almond butter. This blend provides protein, vitamins, and healthy fats that satisfy cravings while supporting joint health and overall nutrition.

Roasted chickpeas mixed with olive oil and your favorite spices, like cumin or paprika, are another satisfying option that will help you feel full in between meals and less likely to reach for less healthy snacks. By paying attention to your cravings and selecting nutrient-dense options, you can keep your diet balanced while managing your arthritis and promoting general well-being.

HEALTHY SOUP RECIPES

Finding soothing soup recipes for arthritis requires choosing ingredients that support joint health as well as comfort. Start with a robust bone broth base that is slowly simmered to extract healthy nutrients like collagen, which supports joint strength and flexibility. Add anti-inflammatory spices like turmeric and ginger, which have been shown to relieve pain. Use blended vegetables, such as sweet potatoes or cauliflower, to add richness without adding dairy, while keeping the soup light and easy to digest.

Try some other combinations, like lentil and spinach soup or chicken and vegetable soup. These are high in protein and fiber, which is good for keeping you energized and supporting your general health. If you want to add flavor without going overboard, use natural herbs like thyme and rosemary, which are also high in antioxidants.

If you stick to nutrient-dense ingredients and season them carefully, you can make soups that are not only filling but also good for your joints.

For healthy, well-balanced salads, try starting with a base of leafy greens, like spinach or kale, which are high in vitamins C and K, which are important for maintaining bone health and lowering inflammation. Then, add colorful veggies, like bell peppers, carrots, and cucumbers, which are high in fiber and antioxidants. Finally, add lean proteins, like grilled chicken or tofu, for muscle support and long-lasting energy.

Add nuts and seeds, like almonds or pumpkin seeds, to enhance flavor and increase nutrient absorption. Nuts and seeds are high in magnesium and omega-3 fatty acids, which help to lubricate joints and relax muscles. Whole grains, like quinoa or brown rice, add complex carbohydrates and extra fiber and give a satisfying crunch.

Toss salads with homemade vinaigrettes made with olive oil, lemon juice, and herbs, like basil or parsley, to create a well-balanced flavor combination without added sugars or preservatives.

SOME ADVICE FOR CREATING ARTHRITIS-FRIENDLY SOUPS

Making soups for people with arthritis requires thoughtful ingredient selection and cooking methods that put joint health and general well-being first. Start with low-sodium broth bases, or make your own to minimize salt intake. Then, add antioxidant- and anti-inflammatory-rich vegetables, like bell peppers, tomatoes, and leafy greens, to help boost immunity and lessen joint pain and stiffness.

You can make soups that are both nutritious and supportive of managing arthritis by using lean proteins like chicken or fish, which provide essential amino acids for muscle repair and strength; avoiding heavy cream-based soups in favor of alternatives like coconut milk or blended vegetables for a creamy texture without dairy;

and utilizing herbs and spices like turmeric, ginger, and garlic, which are known for their anti-inflammatory benefits and ability to enhance flavor without the need for excess salt or unhealthy fats.

DRESSINGS FOR SALADS THAT INCREASE NUTRITION

Adding flavor to salads with healthy dressings means choosing ingredients that are good for the joints as well as taste good. An excellent starting point is an olive oil, which is high in monounsaturated fats that support heart health and reduce inflammation. Vinegar like apple cider or balsamic offers antioxidants and aid in digestion. Finally, fresh herbs like cilantro or basil taste good and provide vitamins and minerals that are important for overall health.

Use natural sweeteners like honey or maple syrup sparingly when making homemade dressings to avoid adding too many calories. Try different citrus juices, like lemon or lime, to add tanginess. Minced garlic or shallots can add depth of flavor and additional anti-inflammatory benefits. By emphasizing nutrient-dense ingredients and exercising mindful portion control, you can make dressings that improve joint health and overall vitality while also boosting the nutritional value of your salads.

INCLUDING VEGETABLES AND GREENS FOR JOINT HEALTH

Including greens and vegetables in your diet for joint health means choosing nutrient-dense foods that offer vital vitamins, minerals, and antioxidants. Start with leafy greens like kale or spinach, which are high in vitamins A, C, and K, which are important for immune system function and bone health. Then, include vibrant veggies like carrots, bell peppers, and broccoli, which offer a variety of antioxidants that help fight oxidative stress and inflammation.

Incorporate cruciferous vegetables, such as Brussels sprouts and cauliflower, which are high in fiber and have anti-inflammatory qualities. These vegetables also aid in digestion and support gut health, which is closely related to joint function.

Try different cooking techniques, like roasting, sautéing, or steaming, to preserve nutrients while enhancing flavors. Add a variety of vegetables to salads, soups, and stir-fries to ensure a diverse array of nutrients that support joint lubrication and mobility. You can optimize your diet for better joint health and general well-being by emphasizing seasonal, fresh produce and careful preparation methods.

HEALTHIER SUBSTITUTES FOR DESSERT

To keep a balanced diet while managing arthritis, it's important to find healthier dessert substitutes. Try desserts that include natural sweeteners like honey or maple syrup, which can help reduce inflammation. Try whole grain and oat-based recipes to add fiber and nutrients.

For example, oatmeal cookies sweetened with mashed bananas and a dash of cinnamon can satisfy a sweet tooth without sending blood sugar levels skyrocketing.

Nuts and seeds give desserts a crunch and provide vital omega-3 fatty acids, which are good for people with arthritis because they reduce inflammation. If you want a healthy, on-the-go snack, try making energy balls with blended dates, nuts, and seeds; they taste great and are good for your joints because they are high in nutrients and low in inflammation.

Desserts like yogurt parfaits layered with fresh berries and a drizzle of dark chocolate are a satisfying treat that's low in added sugars and high in beneficial nutrients. By opting for these healthier alternatives, people with arthritis can enjoy desserts guilt-free while supporting their overall health.

You should also look into desserts that feature antioxidant-rich fruits like berries, which can help combat oxidative stress associated with arthritis.

FRUIT-BASED SWEETS

Fruit-based sweets are great for people with arthritis because they offer natural sweetness along with a range of vitamins and minerals. Fruit salads, which are packed with vitamin C to support joint health and reduce inflammation, are a refreshing dessert option. Another fruit-based idea is to blend frozen bananas with a little almond milk to make a dairy-free, creamy "ice cream" that can be garnished with nuts or seeds for extra texture and nutrition.

Another tasty treat that can be had as a light dessert or snack is grilled fruit skewers. Just skewer pineapple, mango, and peach chunks and grill until caramelized. This brings out their natural sweetness and offers a filling dessert option without the added sugars. Fruit-based desserts taste great and also contain vital nutrients that promote overall health and well-being.

A more decadent option would be to bake fruit crisps or cobblers with whole-grain oats and a small amount of sweetener. These are simple to prepare and can be tailored to your preferred fruits and spices, such as nutmeg or cinnamon.

Increasing the amount of fruit-based treats in your diet will help you enjoy satisfying desserts while managing the symptoms of arthritis and supporting joint health.

RECIPES FOR ARTHRITIS-FRIENDLY DESSERTS: BAKING TIPS

Bakeware and non-stick pans reduce the need for greasing, which can be difficult for people with arthritis.

Additionally, silicone molds are flexible, so you can remove baked goods without straining your hands. These are just a few of the tips and techniques that can help people with arthritis bake more easily.

For mixing and blending, use electric mixers or food processors rather than hand stirrers; these appliances ease joint strain and facilitate smooth batters and doughs; for measuring, use ergonomic measuring cups and spoons with large, comfortable handles to minimize discomfort.

Try experimenting with gluten-free flours such as almond flour or coconut flour, which are kinder to the stomach and may help some people with arthritis feel less irritated. These flours also give baked goods a richer, nutty flavor. To enhance flavor and texture without using a lot of refined sugars, add lots of nuts, seeds, and fruits to your recipes.

Simplifying baking recipes and utilizing arthritis-friendly ingredients can make baking more pleasurable and accessible for people with arthritis, allowing them to continue enjoying homemade delicacies without putting additional strain on their joints.

CONTROLLING SUGAR CONSUMPTION

To lower inflammation and improve overall health, people with arthritis must control their sugar intake. To start, read food labels and select items that have little to no added sugar. Swap out sugary desserts for naturally sweetened options like fresh fruit or yogurt with honey. Gradually cut back on the amount of sugar you add to recipes until your taste buds become accustomed to less sweetness.

Instead of using sugar in baking and cooking, try using low-calorie, non-glycemic sweeteners like stevia or monk fruit extract, which provide a sweet taste without the health risks of consuming too much sugar.

Watch out for hidden sugars in processed foods like sauces, condiments, and packaged snacks. To reduce the amount of added sugar, make homemade versions whenever you can.

Try adding spices like nutmeg, cinnamon, or vanilla extract to foods to bring out their natural sweetness.

Small changes to minimize sugar consumption can have considerable benefits for joint health and inflammation control. People with arthritis can actively manage their sugar intake to enhance their general health and well-being while still enjoying occasional indulgences.

ENJOYING WITHOUT FEELING BAD

Desserts can be enjoyed guilt-free as long as they are chosen wisely and in moderation. Dark chocolate, for example, is high in antioxidants and can help reduce inflammation. You can also occasionally enjoy small portions of your favorite desserts, with the emphasis being on enjoying each bite and savoring the flavors.

When it comes to preventing overindulgence and fostering a healthy relationship with food, practice mindful eating by paying attention to cues of hunger and fullness instead of eating out of habit or emotion.

When it comes to satisfying sweet cravings, go for naturally sweetened options like fruit or homemade treats made with whole ingredients.

Dessert is a normal part of a balanced diet, and it can be enjoyed guilt-free when approached mindfully. To satisfy your sweet tooth while practicing moderation, think about sharing desserts with friends or family so that you can enjoy a taste without consuming a full portion.

People with arthritis can still enjoy sweets and have a nutritious diet at the same time by making thoughtful decisions and in moderation. It's all about fueling your body with nutrient-dense meals and rewarding yourself with the odd dessert as part of a balanced lifestyle.

TIPS ON HYDRATION TO MANAGE ARTHRITIS

Drinking enough water is critical for effectively managing the symptoms of arthritis. Dehydration can worsen joint pain and stiffness, so it's important to stay hydrated throughout the day. Try to drink 8 to 10 glasses of water a day, spread out evenly, to stay hydrated. To add some taste and benefits to your hydration, add slices of citrus fruits, like lemon or orange, or add cucumber and mint for a refreshing twist. Herbal teas and diluted fruit juices can also add to your daily fluid intake. Avoid drinking too much caffeinated and sugary beverages, as they can also dehydrate you.

Together with water, hydrating foods can help you manage your arthritis. High-water foods such as watermelon, cucumber, celery, and strawberries can help you stay hydrated overall. Clear, non-creamy-based soups and broths are also great ways to stay hydrated while getting essential nutrients.

When choosing packaged soups, look for low-sodium options. By emphasizing both fluids and hydrating foods, you can help relieve joint pain and stay healthy overall.

Keeping yourself properly hydrated is an easy yet powerful way to support your arthritis management plan. You can support joint mobility and reduce inflammation by drinking enough fluids and eating foods that are hydrating. Try a variety of flavors and hydration sources to see what works best for you; try to stay consistent throughout the day. Pay attention to your body's thirst signals and adjust your fluid intake as necessary, particularly in warmer weather or when you're exercising. By making hydration a priority, you can improve your general health and well-being while effectively managing your arthritis symptoms.

RECIPES FOR COOL DRINKS

Making tasty drinks that are friendly to arthritis can be a fun way to relieve symptoms. To start, try simple fruit-infused water combinations like lemon and cucumber or berries with mint; these offer antioxidants and vitamins that support joint health in addition to hydration. Another refreshing option is coconut water blended with a splash of pineapple juice and a hint of ginger for a tropical twist; this blend not only hydrates but also provides electrolytes that can help with muscle and joint function.

Smoothies are another great way to combine hydration and nutrition. Blend leafy greens like spinach or kale with fruits like berries or bananas, adding a splash of almond milk or yogurt for creaminess. Optionally, incorporate a scoop of collagen powder for added joint support and protein. For a calming treat, try making herbal iced teas using ingredients like chamomile, which has anti-inflammatory properties, or ginger tea, which is known for its digestive and anti-nausea benefits. These teas can be sweetened with a touch of honey or agave syrup if desired.

Try varying these recipes to see what works best for your diet and taste preferences. By emphasizing hydrating ingredients and avoiding high sugar and caffeine content, you can make drinks that taste great and help you achieve your arthritis management objectives. Sip these revitalizing drinks all day long to stay nourished, hydrated, and energized while supporting joint health and overall well-being.

SMOOTHIES FOR HEALTHY JOINTS

Smoothies are a tasty and easy way to get nutrients that support joint health into your diet. Start with a base of leafy greens like spinach or kale, which are rich in vitamins, minerals, and antioxidants that help reduce inflammation. Add fruits like bananas, which provide potassium and support muscle function, or berries, which are high in antioxidants and have anti-inflammatory properties. For extra protein and joint support, think about adding a scoop of Greek yogurt or collagen powder, both of which support overall joint health and tissue repair.

Blend until smooth and enjoy as a nourishing snack or meal replacement that supports joint mobility and overall well-being. If you would like to add more flavor and nutrients to your smoothie, consider adding ingredients like chia seeds or flaxseeds, which are rich in omega-3 fatty acids that help reduce inflammation. You can also opt to add a splash of almond milk or coconut water for a creamy texture and additional hydration benefits. Tailor your smoothie to your taste preferences and dietary needs, adjusting sweetness with natural sweeteners like honey or dates if desired.

Smoothies can be customized to meet specific nutritional goals, which make them a great choice for people with arthritis. You can improve your overall diet while enjoying nutrient-dense, delicious beverages by adding ingredients that promote joint health and reduce inflammation.

Try different combinations and flavors until you find a smoothie you love, then incorporate it into your daily routine for sustained energy, hydration, and joint support.

The anti-inflammatory effects of chamomile tea, which is well-known for its calming properties, can help reduce joint pain and stiffness. Ginger tea is another great option, as ginger contains compounds that inhibit inflammation and may alleviate arthritis symptoms. Turmeric tea, which is made from the potent spice turmeric, is rich in curcumin, a compound with powerful anti-inflammatory and antioxidant properties that support joint health. Herbal teas are a soothing and flavorful way to support joint health and manage arthritis symptoms naturally.

When preparing herbal teas, consider adding a little honey or lemon for flavor without adding added sugars, enhancing both taste and potential health benefits. Peppermint tea relieves digestive discomfort and has a refreshing taste that can be enjoyed hot or cold. Its menthol content may also help relax muscles and ease tension around joints. Green tea is highly respected for its high antioxidant content, particularly catechins, which have anti-inflammatory effects that may benefit arthritis sufferers.

Warm cups of herbal tea in the morning or evening as part of a soothing ritual, knowing that each sip enhances your general well-being and naturally supports joint health. Adding herbal teas to your daily routine can be a comforting and health-promoting practice for managing arthritis. Try different varieties to find those that suit your palate and offer the most relief from joint discomfort.

ALCOHOL WITH ARTHRITIS: IMPORTANT INFORMATION

To effectively manage symptoms of arthritis, it is important to understand the relationship between alcohol consumption and arthritis. Moderate alcohol consumption may have some cardiovascular benefits, but excessive alcohol consumption can worsen inflammation and contribute to joint pain. Reducing or completely avoiding alcohol consumption can help improve overall health and reduce symptoms of arthritis.

Alcohol can also interact with medications that are frequently prescribed for arthritis, potentially decreasing their effectiveness or causing harmful side effects.

If you choose to drink alcohol, do so in moderation and think about low-alcohol options like wine spritzers or light beer. Pay attention to how alcohol affects your body and how it affects the symptoms of your arthritis. Avoid dehydration by alternating alcoholic beverages with water or other non-alcoholic drinks to minimize joint pain.

Talk to your healthcare provider about your alcohol consumption to make sure it fits with your overall health goals and arthritis management plan.

Making thoughtful decisions about alcohol consumption can contribute to a healthier lifestyle and improved quality of life while living with arthritis. If you experience increased pain or discomfort after drinking, consider reducing your alcohol intake or exploring alternative beverages that support your arthritis management goals.

By understanding the impact of alcohol on arthritis and making informed choices, you can better manage your symptoms and support joint health. Prioritize moderation and hydration while monitoring how alcohol affects your arthritis symptoms.

CHAPTER FIVE

THE BENEFITS OF EXERCISE FOR TREATING ARTHRITIS

Frequent exercise is essential for controlling the symptoms of arthritis and preserving joint health. Low-impact activities like yoga, walking, or swimming help to increase flexibility, strengthen the muscles surrounding the joints, and decrease stiffness. They also improve circulation, which can help to reduce pain and inflammation. Begin with mild movements and increase the intensity gradually as your body adjusts. It's vital to pay attention to your body and avoid exercises that put undue strain on your joints. Including a variety of exercises guarantees that different muscle groups are worked, supporting overall joint function.

Aim for at least 150 minutes of moderate-intensity exercise per week, spread across several sessions. Remember to warm up before exercise and cool down afterward to prevent injury and reduce stiffness.

Strength training exercises help build muscle mass and support joints, reducing the load on them during daily activities. Using resistance bands or light weights can improve strength without putting excessive strain on joints. Flexibility exercises like stretching or tai chi increase the range of motion and joint mobility, easing arthritis symptoms.

Regular physical activity helps manage weight, which lessens stress on joints and lowers the risk of developing other health conditions. It also improves mood and general well-being. By incorporating exercise into your routine, you can effectively manage the symptoms of arthritis and enhance your quality of life.

TECHNIQUES FOR STRESS MANAGEMENT

Because stress exacerbates pain and inflammation, it is critical to managing stress to effectively treat arthritis. Practicing mindfulness techniques to stay present and focused can help reduce anxiety and improve coping mechanisms. Making time for hobbies or other enjoyable activities can also help reduce stress and promote relaxation. Stress management techniques include deep breathing exercises, meditation, and progressive muscle relaxation.

Establish a routine that includes adequate rest to support overall well-being. Recognize triggers that cause stress and develop strategies to minimize their impact on your daily life.

Regular physical activity, such as walking or yoga, not only benefits joints but also helps alleviate stress. Engage in activities that promote relaxation, such as spending time in nature or listening to calming music.

Practicing mindfulness and relaxation techniques regularly can help you lower stress levels, improve your emotional well-being, and manage arthritis-related challenges. By incorporating stress management techniques into your daily routine, you can improve your overall quality of life and cope better with the symptoms of arthritis.

THE EFFECT OF SLEEP ON ARTHRITIS SYMPTOMS

Being able to get a good night's sleep is crucial for managing the symptoms of arthritis because it promotes healing and reduces inflammation. You can help your body regulate its internal clock by creating a sleep-friendly environment in your bedroom by keeping it cool, dark, and quiet. You can also promote relaxation by limiting screen time and avoiding heavy meals and caffeine right before bed.

Before going to bed, use techniques for relaxing the mind and body, such as progressive muscle relaxation or deep breathing. You can also incorporate gentle stretching exercises or a warm bath to help relax muscles and relieve tension.

To support painful joints and ensure that you are in a comfortable sleeping position, use pillows or cushions. If pain or discomfort interferes with your ability to sleep, speak with your healthcare provider about pain management options or medications that can help you sleep better.

Resolving sleep disruptions is essential to effectively managing the symptoms of arthritis. By making sleep hygiene a priority and implementing relaxing techniques, you may improve the quality of your sleep, lessen pain and inflammation, and boost your general health and well-being.

INCLUDING MINDFULNESS IN EVERYDAY ACTIVITIES

Including mindfulness practices like yoga, deep breathing exercises, or meditation in your daily routine can help reduce stress, anxiety, and pain associated with arthritis. Start with short sessions and gradually increase duration as you become more comfortable with the practice. Mindfulness is defined as being present in the moment and non-judgmentally aware of thoughts, emotions, and sensations.

Engage in mindful activities, like walking or gardening, by focusing on each movement and sensation. This can increase awareness of body mechanics and reduce strain on joints during daily activities. Practice mindful eating by paying attention to flavors, textures, and sensations while eating. This helps cultivate a healthy relationship with food and promotes mindful choices that support overall well-being.

Practicing mindfulness regularly can help you develop a better feeling of acceptance and awareness, which supports the successful management of your arthritis. It also helps you become more emotionally resilient, improve your coping mechanisms, and live a higher quality of life overall.

LONG-TERM PLANS FOR EATING A BALANCED DIET

Incorporating anti-inflammatory foods like fatty fish, nuts, seeds, and olive oil can help reduce inflammation and alleviate arthritis symptoms. Limit processed foods, sugary beverages, and foods high in saturated fats, as they can exacerbate symptoms. Eating a variety of nutrient-dense foods, such as fruits, vegetables, whole grains, lean proteins, and healthy fats, is essential for managing arthritis symptoms and supporting overall health.

Plan meals that are balanced and portion-controlled to maintain a healthy weight, which reduces stress on joints. Consider consulting with a registered dietitian who specializes in arthritis to develop a personalized meal plan that meets your nutritional needs and supports your goals for managing your arthritis. Drink plenty of water throughout the day to support joint function and overall health.

To create long-lasting habits that support health and well-being, gradually modify your diet while keeping an eye on how your body reacts to various foods, and make necessary dietary adjustments to optimize arthritis management. By following a healthy eating pattern and making well-informed food choices, you can support joint health, reduce inflammation, and enhance your overall quality of life.

CHAPTER SIX

HANDLING WEIGHT WHEN YOU HAVE ARTHRITIS

A balanced diet rich in fruits, vegetables, lean proteins, and whole grains is an effective way to help maintain a healthy weight. It's also important to watch portion sizes and avoid excessive calorie intake, as excess weight can exacerbate arthritis symptoms. Managing weight is important when you have arthritis because it reduces stress on your joints and improves overall mobility and pain management.

Apart from diet, consistent physical activity plays a crucial role in weight management and joint health enhancement. Low-impact activities such as walking, swimming, or cycling can assist you in staying active without causing undue strain on your joints. Speak with a physical therapist or your healthcare provider to create an exercise regimen that is safe and appropriate for your condition.

It's important to note that slow weight loss is crucial, as sudden weight changes can aggravate arthritis symptoms.

In addition, drinking plenty of water supports overall bodily functions and helps maintain joint lubrication; limiting alcohol and sugary drinks can also help reduce unnecessary calorie intake; and when you combine these three factors—a balanced diet, regular exercise, and adequate hydration—you can effectively manage your weight and alleviate the symptoms of arthritis.

STRATEGIES FOR EATING OUT

When you have arthritis, eating out can be difficult, but there are some strategies you can use to enjoy meals outside of your home while managing your condition: first, look for restaurants that offer healthy options and can accommodate special dietary requirements; many restaurants now have nutritional information available or have low-sodium or heart-healthy menu items.

To curb portion sizes and avoid overindulging, choose grilled, baked, or steamed dishes when placing your order rather than fried ones, which are frequently heavy in unhealthy fats. You can also ask for sauces and dressings to be served on the side to help you keep portion sizes under control.

Ask questions about ingredients, cooking techniques, and substitutions to meet your dietary restrictions. Many restaurants are willing to accommodate special requests, such as preparing dishes without certain ingredients or modifying recipes to suit your needs. Communicating with restaurant staff is essential.

Finally, eat slowly and appreciate each bite to feel satiated without going overboard. By planning and making educated decisions, you may dine out while efficiently managing your arthritis and maintaining a balanced diet. Pay attention to your body's hunger cues and be cautious of portion sizes.

When it comes to managing your diet, especially when it comes to managing arthritis, it is important to understand food labels. Look at the serving size first, as this is the portion on which all nutritional information is based. Then, pay attention to the calories per serving and determine whether the food fits into your daily calorie intake goals.

Next, review the ingredient list. Foods high in saturated fats, trans fats, sodium, and added sugars can aggravate arthritis symptoms and cause inflammation. Ingredients are listed in descending order of weight, so the first few ingredients make up the majority of the product.

Look for foods labeled as low-sodium, low-fat, or high-fiber, which can support joint health and overall well-being. Concentrate on nutrient-dense foods that provide essential vitamins, minerals, and antioxidants. Knowing what's on food labels enables you to make healthier decisions that can help manage arthritis symptoms and improve overall health.

Keeping a food journal to monitor how specific foods impact your symptoms is one way to manage dietary restrictions in conjunction with arthritis. Start by identifying foods that worsen arthritis symptoms or cause inflammation, such as processed foods, red meat, and foods high in sugar or saturated fats.

Speak with a registered dietitian or other healthcare professional to create a customized meal plan that satisfies your nutritional requirements and stays away from trigger foods. They can also assist you in finding other nutrient sources and guarantee that your diet is balanced to promote joint health and general well-being.

Try to incorporate anti-inflammatory foods (fatty fish, nuts, seeds, and colorful fruits and vegetables) into your daily meals while gradually reducing or eliminating foods that aggravate your symptoms. By taking proactive measures to manage dietary restrictions, you can maximize your health and well-being even with arthritis.

A change in diet can help effectively manage pain and inflammation during flare-ups of arthritis. Anti-inflammatory foods, like leafy greens, berries, olive oil, and turmeric, have properties that can help reduce swelling and discomfort. Foods high in refined sugars, processed foods, and alcohol are examples of trigger foods that may exacerbate symptoms.

Drink plenty of water throughout the day to help flush out toxins and reduce inflammation. You can also incorporate herbal teas or antioxidant-rich beverages to further promote joint health. Stay hydrated to maintain joint lubrication and support general biological processes.

Speaking with your healthcare provider or a nutritionist can offer guidance on modifying your diet during flare-ups to effectively manage symptoms. Additionally, pay attention to changes in symptoms and make modifications as needed, such as reducing portion sizes or temporarily eliminating certain foods.

Finally, listen to your body and modify your diet based on how you feel.

You may lessen pain, inflammation, and suffering during arthritis flare-ups by taking proactive measures with your diet, which will enable you to continue leading a more active and healthy lifestyle.

www.ingramcontent.com/pod-product-compliance
Lightning Source LLC
Chambersburg PA
CBHW050651250726
48662CB00002B/607